DASH DIET

A Complete Step By Step Beginners Guide

The best diet, the best diet for diabetes, the healthiest diet and so on…these are just some of the attributes given to the DASH diet. Makes one wonder what it is about DASH diet that has gotten it so much praise by the medical society!

The DASH diet has proven to be effective for a number of ailments including high blood pressure, cholesterol, diabetes, kidney stones, heart diseases and many others. One common misperception about DASH diet is that it is for people having the above mentioned diseases only. Well, this is just a small definition of this vast term.

The health benefits of DASH diet stated in this book are proof enough of the fact that DASH diet is for everyone. This guide tells you how this form of diet is helpful in staying healthy. From the basic nutritional DASH guidelines to a step by step DASH procedure and an easy-to-follow 7 day DASH diet plan, this book tells you all you need to know about DASH diet.

So don't just stop here. Keep on reading and find the DASH secrets of staying healthy.

Table of Contents

Fully read as 'Dietary Approaches to Stop Hypertension', DASH is a form of diet that is proven to be very effective in the treatment of high blood pressure and high cholesterol.

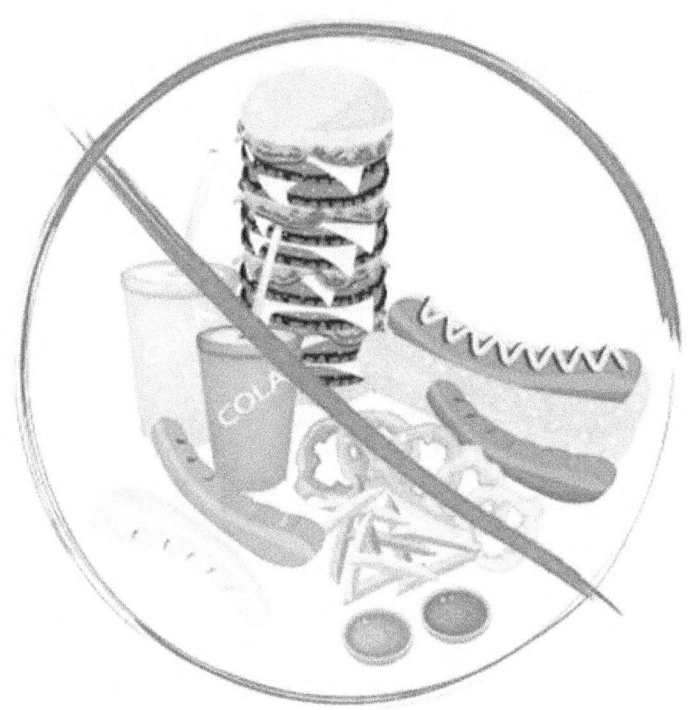

The normal level of blood pressure among adults is 120/80 mmHg. Even a slight increase in the blood pressure above the normal numbers is unhealthy and poses greater health risks.

Several studies have been conducted so far and all of them have ended up in favor of DASH diet. One such study was conducted by National Heart, Lung, and Blood Institute (NHLBI). According the findings of the mentioned research, blood pressures can be reduced and then maintained by following a diet plan that is low in bad cholesterol and saturated fats, and high in fruits, grains, vegetables and fat free dairy products.

A basic DASH diet plan can be described as follows.

1. It includes nuts, chicken, fish and other whole grain products.

2. It contains almost no amount of white sugars and other sugary drinks.

3. It is rich in minerals such as potassium, magnesium, protein and calcium.

The above mentioned attributes of DASH diet are vindicated by the following table. It represents the daily nutritional goals that were used in the DASH studies.

Cholesterol	150 mg
Sodium	2,300 mg
Potassium	4,700 mg
Calcium	1,250 mg
Magnesium	500 mg
Fiber	30 g
Total fat	27% of calories
Saturated fat	6% of calories
Protein	18% of calories
Carbohydrate	55% of calories

Note: These guidelines are based on 2,000 calorie eating plan.

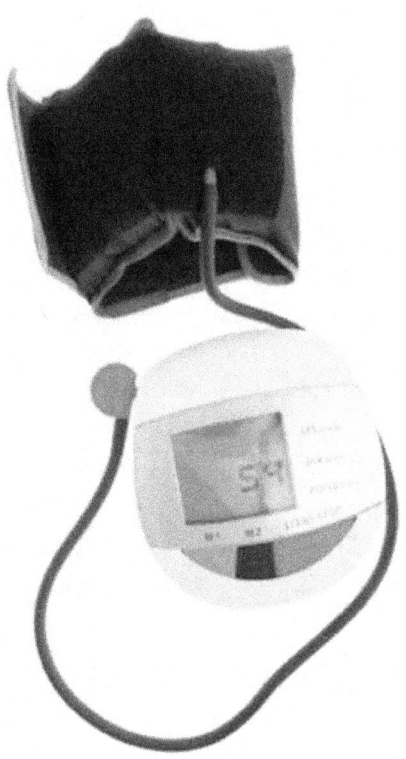

Though DASH diet is for everyone, it specifically addresses and is extremely beneficial for people having high blood pressure. So the next step after knowing the basics of DASH diet is to check your blood pressure.

But what actually is meant by this term. Also known as hypertension, blood pressure in its simplest form, is the pressure that the blood exerts against our artery walls.

The level of hypertension is based on two statistics, namely systolic pressure and diastolic pressure. The former represents the blood pressure when the heart beats, whereas the latter is recorded when the heart relaxes between beats. Both the numbers are recorded in millimeters of mercury (mmHg).

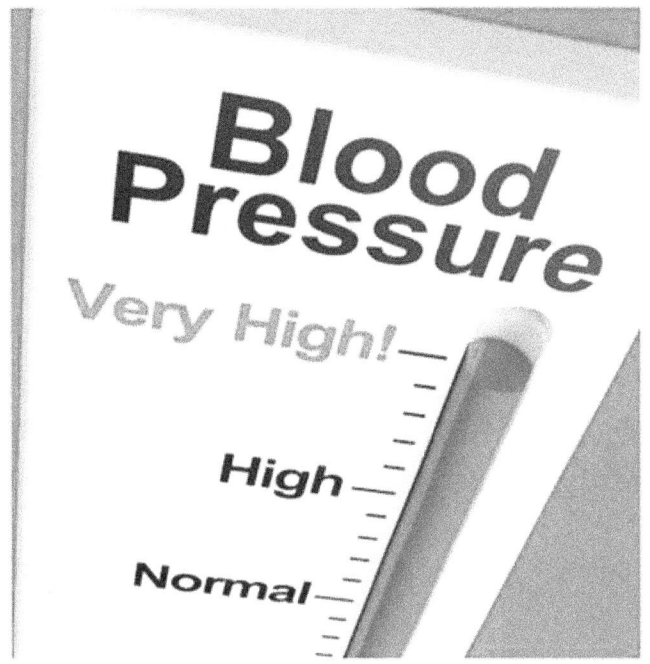

The standard levels of blood pressure are divided into three categories, as stated below.

1. Systolic pressure: **<120**

   Diastolic pressure: **<80**

It is a good sign if your blood pressure lies below the above mentioned statistics. It means you have normal blood pressure.

2. Systolic pressure: **120 - 139**

   Diastolic pressure: **80 – 89**

The above mentioned blood pressure levels are a sign of Pre-hypertension. If not controlled at this stage, it could lead to high blood pressure.

3. Systolic pressure: **> 140**

   Diastolic pressure: **> 90**

These levels indicate Hypertension, means high blood pressure.

Notes:

i.   The above mentioned statistics are standard levels of blood pressure in adults over 18 years who do not have any severe ailment.

ii. The statistics may vary if you have diabetes or any other major illness.

iii. The blood pressure levels also vary according to the age.

iv. If the systolic and diastolic pressure lies in different categories, then the overall status lies in the higher category.

v.   In either case, consult your doctor to know the interpretation of your blood pressure levels.

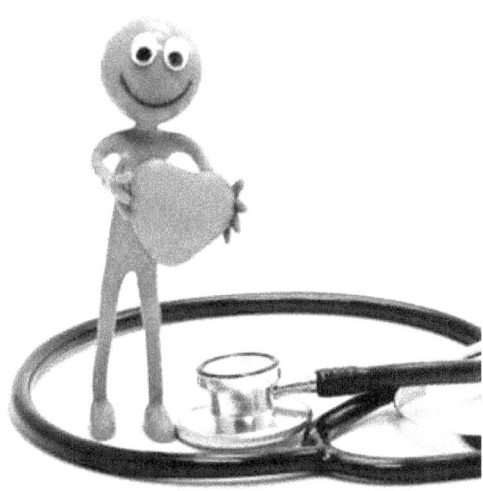

DASH diet has numerous health benefits, not only for those suffering from any major illness but also for perfectly healthy people.

DASH Diet:

i. Lowers blood pressure

ii. Lowers bad cholesterol

iii. Reduces the risk of several types of cancer

iv. Lower the risk of heart disease, heart stroke and heart failure

v. Reduced the chances of developing kidney stones

vi. Lessen the risk of diabetes

vii. Slows down the progression of kidney disease

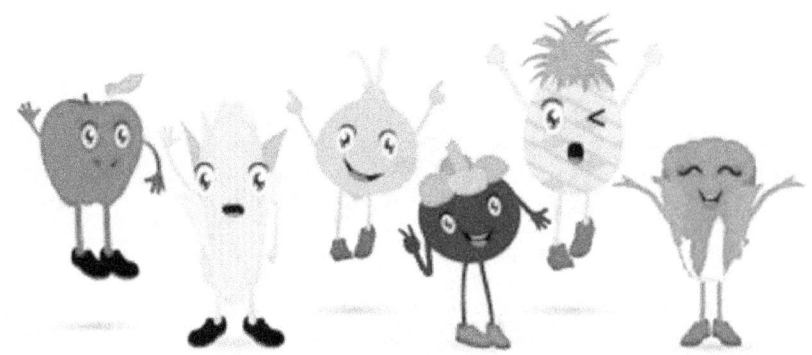

According to the findings of research conducted at the Pennington Biomedical Research Center, the extra intake of fruits, whole grains and vegetables in DASH diet creates plenty of food compounds like   lycopene, beta carotene and isoflavones in the human body. These compounds are known to reduce and control several types of chronic diseases.

DASH diet is quite easy to follow. It is unlike other type of boring and tasteless diets that restrain you to eat almost everything. Before we move on to the step by step process of DASH diets, let's give you a brief idea of what this diet contains.

You will be required to do the following when following a DASH diet. Well you don't have to jump to the DASH eating habits immediately. Go gradually taking one step at a time.

i. If you don't eat fruit at all or take fruit juices only, then it is time to add two servings of fruit in your daily meals. You can take them anytime you want during the entire day.

ii. If currently you are eating one or two vegetables a day, add two more in your daily serving; one at lunch and another at dinner.

iii. Read the nutritional information on any product that you intend to buy. Compare it with the nutritional information of others products of the same type and select the one having the lowest amount of saturated fat and trans fat.

iv. The DASH diet requires you to consume fat free or one percent fat dairy products at least three times a day.

v. Limit the amount of lean meat to 6 ounces per day, maximum 3 ounces at a time.

vi. Make a habit of having at least two fully vegetarian meals per week.

vii. The DASH diet requires you to increase the consumption of fruits, vegetables, whole wheat pasta, brown rice and cooked dry beans.

viii. DASH diet does not ask you to close your eyes when passing through the snack rack on Wal-Mart. Pick low fat snacks such as nuts, graham crackers, low-fat yogurt, unsalted rice cakes and unsalted popcorn. These will fulfill your appetite for snacks.

Note: You don't have to adopt all these eating habits at once. Take one at a time. For example, gradually increase your consumption of dairy products. Once you are comfortable with this eating pattern, move on the next.

Now that you have an idea on what it takes to adopt a DASH diet plan, let's move on to the step by step procedure.

Step 1: How Much Do You Need?

The first step is to estimate your calorie needs according to your age, gender and activity level. The red table is for women and the blue table indicates the standard calorie needs for men.

Age (years)	Calories According To The Activity Level		
	Sedentary	Moderate	Active
19-30	2,000	2,000 - 2,200	2,400
31-50	1,800	2,000	2,200
51+	1,600	1,800	2,000 - 2,200

Age (years)	Calories According To The Activity Level		
	Sedentary	Moderate	Active
19-30	2,400	2,600 - 2,800	3,000
31-50	2,200	2,400 - 2,600	2,800 - 3,000
51+	2,000	2,200 - 2,400	2,400 - 2,800

Step 2: How Much You Should Eat?

Once you figured out your calorie needs, the next step is to determine how much you should eat to fulfill your estimated calorie needs.

Look at the table below and see which level of calorie is closest to yours.

Food Category	CALORIES				
	1,600	1,800	2,600	2,000	3,100
	Serving Size				
Grains (mostly whole grains)	6	6	6 - 8	10 - 11	12 - 13
Fat-free or 1-percent dairy products (mostly milk)	2-3	2 - 3	2 - 3	3	3 - 4
Nuts, seeds and legumes	3- 4/ week	4/ week	5/ week	1	1
Vegetables	3 - 4	4 - 5	4 - 5	5 - 6	6
Fruits	4	4 - 5	4 - 5	5 - 6	6
Lean meats, poultry and fish	< 5	< 6	< 7	< 7	6 - 9
Fats and oils	2	2 - 3	2 - 3	3	4
Sweets and added sugars	< 3/ week	< 5/ week	< 5/ week	< 3	< 3
Maximum consumption of sodium/salt (mg/day)	2,300	2,300	2,300	2,300	2,300

The serving quantities are on daily basis unless stated otherwise.

This table gives you an approximate number of servings that you should eat from each food category. Suppose your estimated calorie needs are close to 1,800. It means should consume 6 servings of grains, 4-5 servings of vegetables daily and so on.

Step 3: What You Should Eat?

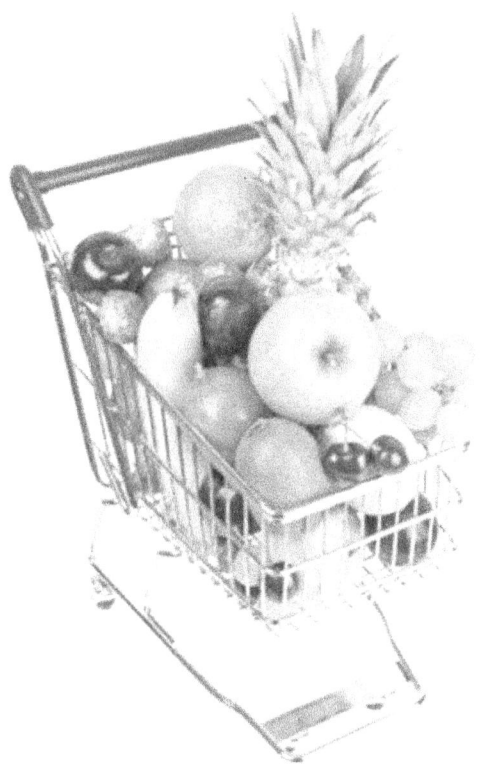

The final step is to determine what you should actually eat. Continuing the example stated in the step 2, if you are supposed to consume 6 servings of grain, then what actually makes up those 6 servings.

This section tells you the serving size, foods that fall in the particular food category and the benefits of the mentioned food items.

Considering the information detailed forward, 6 servings of grain includes 6 slices bread or 6 ounce dry cereals or 3 cups of brown rice or the combination of the three in a proportion that makes total 6 servings.

Grains

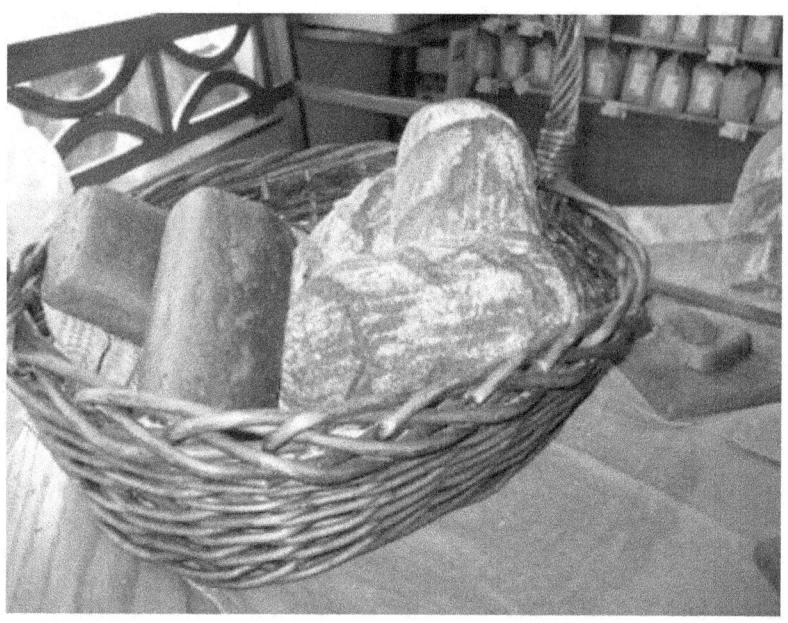

Serving Size

1 slice bread

1 ounce dry cereals

½ cup cooked rice or pasta (Whole Wheat Pasta and Brown rice preferred)

Food Items That Fall In This Category

Whole-wheat bread

Whole Wheat Pasta

Whole-wheat rolls

Pita bread

Whole Wheat bagels

Oatmeal

Unsalted pretzels

Brown rice

Unsalted popcorn without butter

Why Should You Eat It?

Whole grains are abundant in fiber which creates energy in the body.

Fat-Free or One Percent Dairy Products

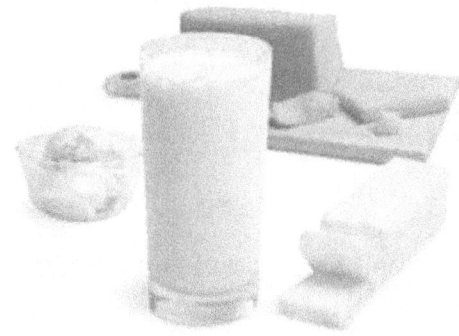

Serving Size

1 cup milk or yogurt

1½ oz cheese

Food Items That Fall In This Category

Fat free milk

Low fat buttermilk

Low fat or fat free yoghurt

Low fat or fat free cheese

Why Should You Eat It?

Dairy products are a major source of calcium and protein. If you are lactose intolerant, then try lactose free milk, soy milk and lactase enzyme pills.

Nuts, Seeds and Legumes

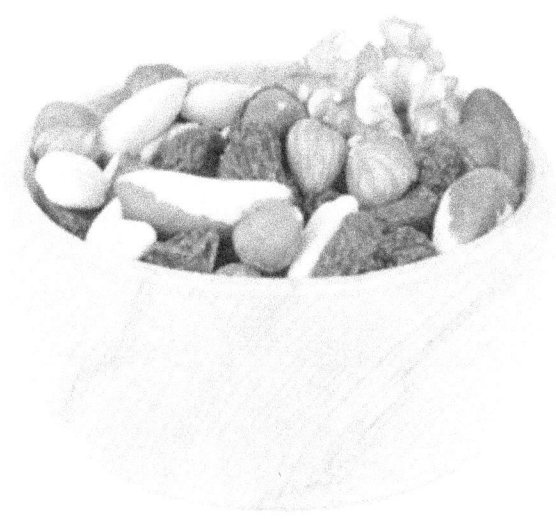

Serving Size

One-third Cup nuts

Half ounce seeds

2 tablespoons peanut butter

Half cup cooked legumes such dried beans, peas etcetera

Food Items That Fall In This Category

Almonds

Mixed nuts

Walnuts

Filberts

Split peas

Sunflower seeds

Peanut butter

Peanuts

Kidney beans

Lentils

Why Should You Eat It?

Nuts, Seeds and Legumes are quite abundant in magnesium, protein and fiber.

Vegetables

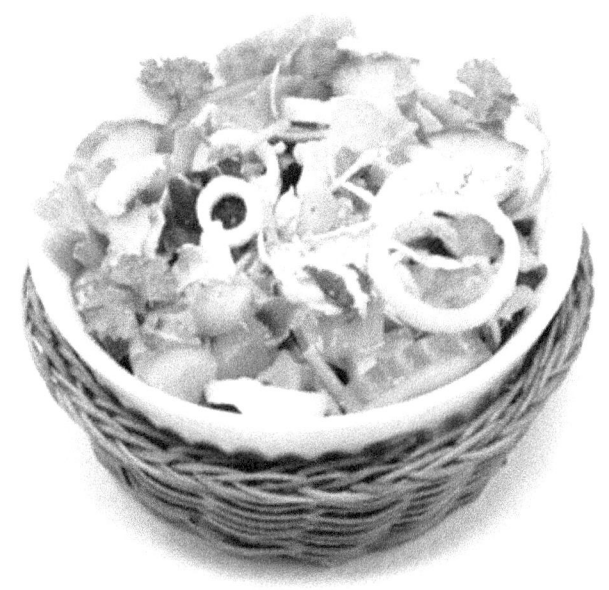

Serving Size

1 cup raw leafy vegetables

Half cup vegetable juice

Half cup cooked vegetables

Food Items That Fall In This Category

Spinach

Carrots

Broccoli

Collards

Green beans

Squash

Lima beans

Green peas

Potatoes

Kale

Lettuce Leaves

Sweet potatoes

Tomatoes

Why Should You Eat It?

Vegetables are rich in magnesium, protein and fiber.

Fruits

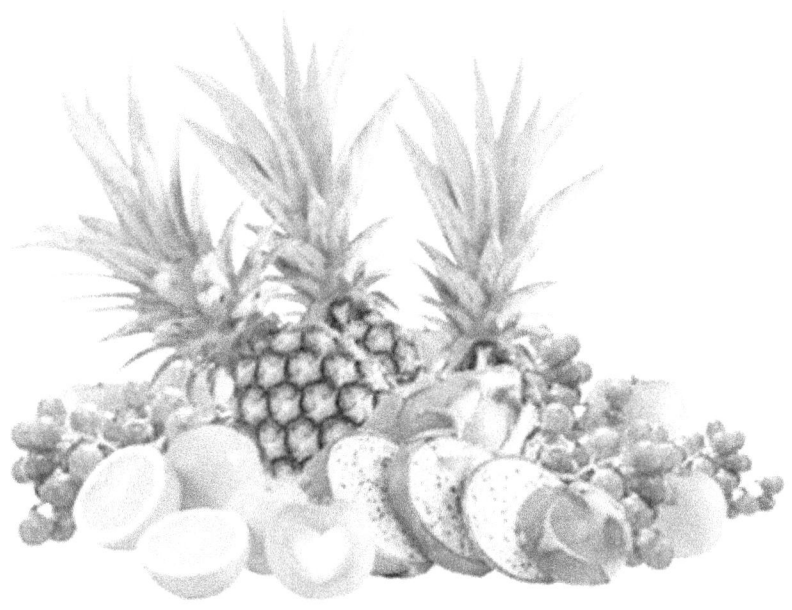

Serving Size

1 fresh fruit

One-fourth cup dried fruit

Half cup fruit juice

Half cup cut-up fresh, frozen, or canned fruit

Food Items That Fall In This Category

Grapes

Oranges

Apples

Dates

Grapefruit / Grapefruit Juice

Apricots

Bananas

Oranges / Orange Juice

Mangoes

Strawberries

Peaches

Sweet Melon

Watermelon

Pineapples

Papaya

Why Should You Eat It?

Fruits are a major source of energy and minerals like protein, magnesium and fiber.

Lean Meats, Poultry and Fish

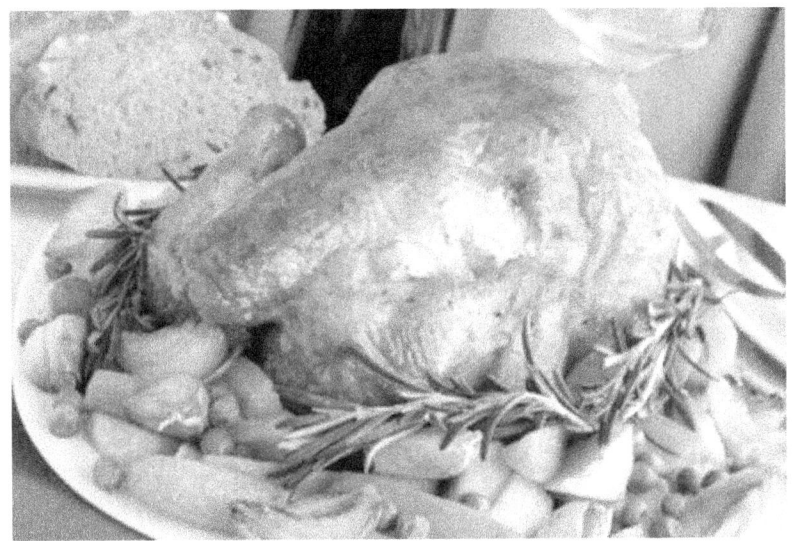

Serving Size

1 ounce cooked meat (Mostly chicken and fish)

1 egg

Food Items That Fall In This Category

Lean meat (cut away the visible fats)

Broiled, grilled, baked, boiled meat

Skinless meat

Why Should You Eat It?

Lean meat provides protein, magnesium and several other minerals.

Fats and Oils

Serving Size

1 teaspoon soft margarine

1 tablespoon mayonnaise

1 teaspoon vegetable oil

2 tablespoon fat free salad dressing

Food Items That Fall In This Category

Vegetable oil

Olive Oil

Canola Oil

Corn Oil

Safflower Oil,

Soft margarine

Low fat mayonnaise

Fat free salad dressing

Why Should You Eat It?

The oils mentioned above are good for lowering blood pressure and cholesterol.

Sweets and Added Sugars

Serving Size

1 tablespoon sugar

Half cup sorbet

1 tablespoon sugar free fruit jelly/ jam

1 cup lemonade

Food Items That Fall In This Category

Fruit flavored gelatin

Sugar free fruit punch

Sugar free hard candy

Maple syrup

Why Should You Eat It?

It satisfies your sweet tooth and fulfills the appetite for deserts. This will help you maintain the DASH diet for a longer span of time.

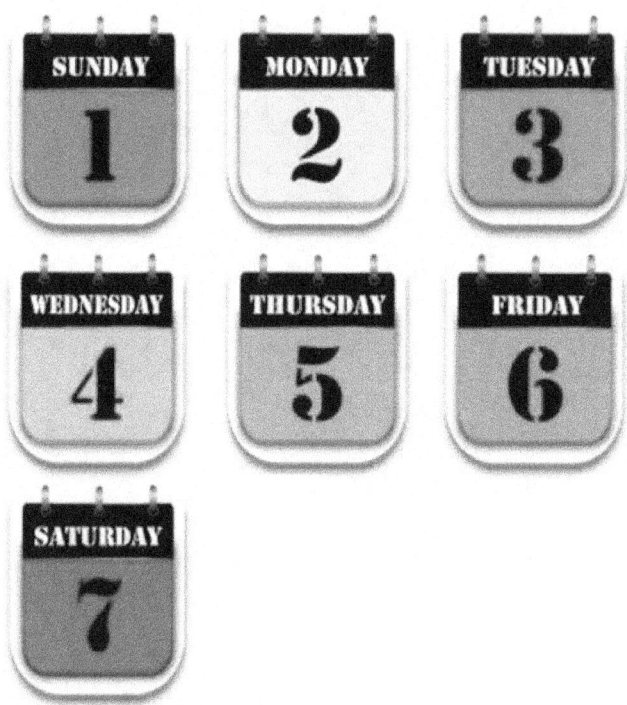

Here comes the most awaited and important part of this guide, the 7 day DASH diet plan. While we have given you several tips on how to adopt a DASH diet, this section presents a detailed seven day DASH plan.

Day 1

Breakfast

1 low fat granola bar

1 banana

Half cup fat free fruit yogurt

1 cup orange juice

1 cup low fat milk

Lunch

Turkey breast sandwich; use the following ingredients to make the sandwich:

3 ounce turkey breast

2 slices whole wheat bread

2 slices tomato

1 large leaf romaine lettuce

2 teaspoon low fat mayonnaise

1 tablespoon Dijon mustard

1 cup steamed broccoli

1 fresh orange

Snacks

2 tablespoon unsalted peanuts

1/4 cup dried apricots

1 cup low fat milk

Dinner

Spicy baked fish (Recipe at the end of this day's plan)

1 cup brown rice

1/4 cups chopped scallions (You can also mix them with brown rice)

Half cup spinach stir friend in 2 teaspoon canola oil

1 tablespoon unsalted almonds

1 cup baby carrots

1 small whole wheat roll with 1 teaspoon soft margarine spread

1 small cookie (preferably sugar free)

Recipe of Spicy Baked Fish

1 lb salmon fillet

1 tablespoon olive oil

1 teaspoon salt free spicy seasoning

1. Preheat oven to 350 °F.

2. Marinate the fish with oil and seasoning

3. Bake it in the preheated oven for 15 minutes

Day 2

Breakfast

1 slice whole wheat bread with 1 teaspoon soft margarine

1 cup fat free fruit yogurt

1 peach

Half cup grape juice

Lunch

Ham sandwich; use the following ingredients to make the sandwich:

    2 ounce low fat, low sodium ham

    2 slices whole wheat bread

    1 slice natural cheddar cheese, low fat

    1 large romaine lettuce leaf

    2 slices tomato

    1 tablespoon mayonnaise, low-fat

1 cup carrot sticks / baby carrots

Snacks

1/3 cup unsalted almonds

1/4 cup dried apricots

1 cup apple juice

1 cup low fat milk

Dinner

Chick 'n' Spanish rice (Recipe at the end of this day's plan)

1 cup green peas; stir fry the peas in 1 teaspoon canola oil

1 cup cantaloupe chunks

1 cup low fat milk

Recipe of Chick 'n' Spanish rice

1 cup chopped onions

3/4 cup green peppers

2 teaspoon vegetable oil

1 8 oz tomato sauce

1 teaspoon chopped parsley

Half teaspoon black pepper

1 teaspoon minced garlic

5 cups cooked brown rice (Boil in plain water without salt)

3 cups skinless chicken breasts, cooked and diced

1. Heat oil in a pan over medium heat

2. Stir fry the onions and green peppers in the oil for 5 minutes

3. Add tomato sauce, parsley, black pepper and minced garlic. Stir for 3 minutes.

4. Add cooked rice and chicken.

5. Stir lightly for 5 minutes.

Day 3

Breakfast

1 cup whole grain oat rings cereal with 1 cup low fat milk

1 banana

1 medium sized raisin bagel

1 tablespoon peanut butter

1 cup orange juice

Lunch

Half cup tuna salad (Recipe at the end of this day's plan)

1 slice whole wheat bread

1 cup cucumber slices

Half cup tomato wedges

1 tablespoon vinaigrette dressing (You can also add the dressing in the cucumber slices or wedges)

Half cup low fat cottage cheese

Half cup canned pineapple

1 tablespoon unsalted almonds

Snacks

1 cup fat free fruit yogurt

2 tablespoon unsalted sunflower seeds

Dinner

3 ounce turkey meatloaf (Recipe at the end of this day's plan)

1 small baked potato; use the following ingredients to make the baked potato.

   1 tablespoon fat free sour cream

   1 tablespoon natural cheddar cheese, fat free or reduced fat

   1 tablespoon chopped scallions

1 cup collard greens stir fried in 1 teaspoon canola oil

1 small whole wheat roll

1 medium peach

Recipe of Tuna Salad

6 ounce canned tuna

Half cup chopped raw celery

1/3 cup chopped green onions

1 large romaine lettuce leaf, shred in a few pieces

6 tablespoon low fat mayonnaise

1. Break tuna with a fork.

2. Add the remaining ingredients and mix well.

Recipe of Turkey Meatloaf

1 lb lean ground turkey

Half cup dry oats

1 egg

1 tablespoon dehydrated flakes of onion,

1/4 cup ketchup

1. Preheat the oven at 350 ˚F

2. Mix well all the ingredients

3. Bake in a loaf pan for 25 minutes

4. Cut into pieces or slices

Day 4

Breakfast

3/4 cup bran flakes cereal

Add 1 medium sized banana in the cereals

Take it with 1 cup fat free/ low fat milk

1 slice whole wheat bread with 1 teaspoon spread of soft margarine

1 cup orange juice

Lunch

Beef sandwich; use the following ingredients to make the beef sandwich:

2 ounce beef

1 tablespoon barbeque sauce

1 large leaf romaine lettuce

1 hamburger bun

2 slices natural cheddar cheese, low fat

2 slices tomato

1 cup potato salad (Recipe at the end of this day's plan)

1 fresh orange

Snacks

1 cup fat free fruit yogurt

1 tablespoon unsalted sunflower seeds

1 tablespoon peanut butter

2 large graham cracker rectangles

Dinner

3 ounce cooked cod fish.

Squeeze 1 teaspoon lemon juice on Cod fish

Half cup boiled brown rice

1 cup spinach, stir fry the spinach in the following ingredients:

1 teaspoon canola oil

1 tablespoon crushed almonds

1 small cornbread muffin with 1 teaspoon soft margarine spread

Recipe of Potato Salad

15 small sized potatoes

1/4 cup green onions, chopped

2 tablespoon olive oil

1 teaspoon dried dill weed

1/4 tsp black pepper

1. Boil potatoes until the soften

2. Let them cool for a while

3. Cut potatoes in small cubes.

4. Stir fry in olive oil with the remaining ingredients.

Day 5

Breakfast

3/4 cup bran flakes cereal

Add 1 medium sized banana in the cereals

Take it with 1 cup fat free/ low fat milk

1 slice whole wheat bread with 1 teaspoon spread of soft margarine

1 cup orange juice

Lunch

3/4 cup chicken salad (of the following ingredients)

Chicken cubes

Lemon juice

Celery

Onion Powder

Pinch of Salt

Fat free mayonnaise

2 slices whole wheat bread with 1 tablespoon Dijon mustard spread

Half cup cucumber slices

1 tablespoon sunflower seeds (You can also add the seeds in the salad)

Half cup tomato wedges

Snacks

1/3 cup unsalted almonds

Half cup fat free fruit yogurt

1/4 cup raisins

Dinner

3 ounce cooked beef

2 tablespoon fat free beef gravy

1 cup green beans, stir fry the beans in the half teaspoon canola oil

1 small baked potato; use the following ingredients to make the baked potato.

1 tablespoon fat free sour cream

1 tablespoon natural cheddar cheese, fat free or reduced fat

1 tablespoon chopped scallions

1 small whole wheat roll with 1 tsp teaspoon soft margarine spread

1 small apple

1 cup low fat or fat free milk

Day 6

Breakfast

1 cup whole grain oat rings

1 banana

1 cup fat free fruit yogurt

1 cup low fat milk

Lunch

Tuna sandwich; use the following ingredients to make the sandwich:

1/2 cup canned tuna

1 large leaf romaine lettuce

1 tablespoon low fat mayonnaise

2 slices tomato

2 slices whole wheat bread

1 medium apple

1 cup low fat milk

Snacks

Half cup unsalted almonds

1/4 cup dry apricots

6 whole wheat crackers

Dinner

Zucchini lasagna (Recipe at the end of this day's plan)

Salad (of the following ingredients)

 1 cup fresh spinach leaves

 1 cup tomato wedges

 2 tablespoon croutons

 1 tablespoon vinaigrette dressing

 1 tablespoon sunflower seeds

1 small whole wheat roll with 1 teaspoon soft margarine

1 cup grape juice

Recipe of the Zucchini Lasagna

1/2 lb lasagna noodles (boil in unsalted water)

3/4 cup low fat grated mozzarella cheese

1 cup fat free cottage cheese

1/4 cup grated Parmesan cheese

2 cups sliced raw zucchini

2 cups low sodium tomato sauce

2 teaspoon dried basil

2 teaspoon dried oregano

1/4 cup chopped onion

1 clove garlic

Pinch of black pepper

1. Preheat oven to 350 °F.

2. Mix well half of the mozzarella cheese and 1 tablespoon Parmesan cheese. Set it aside.

3. In another bowl, mix the remaining mozzarella cheese, Parmesan cheese and all the cottage cheese. Set it aside.

4. Mix tomato sauce with all the other remaining ingredients except zucchini.

5. Spread a fine layer of tomato sauce at the bottom of a baking dish.

6. Spread one third of the lasagna noodles in a single layer on top of the sauce.

7. Add half of the cottage cheese mixture on it.

8. Spread a layer of zucchini

9. Repeat the same layering process two more times.

10. Top it up with the first mixture of cheese

11. Cover the pan with aluminum foil and put in the preheated oven 30 for 40 minutes.

Day 7

Breakfast

Half cup instant oatmeal

1 whole wheat bagel with 1 tablespoon peanut butter spread

1 banana

1 cup low fat milk

Lunch

Chicken breast sandwich; the sandwich should be made of the following ingredients:

3 ounce skinless chicken breast

2 slices whole wheat bread

1 slice natural cheddar cheese, low fat

1 large romaine lettuce leaf

2 slices tomato

1 tablespoon low fat mayonnaise

1 cup cantaloupe chunks

1 cup apple juice

Snacks

1/3 cup unsalted almonds

1/4 cup dried apricots

1 cup fat free fruit yogurt

Dinner

1 cup spaghetti; should be made of the following ingredients:

3/4 cup vegetarian spaghetti sauce (Recipe at the end of this day's plan)

3 tablespoon Parmesan cheese

Spinach salad; Use the following ingredients to make the salad

1 cup fresh spinach leaves

1/4 cup fresh grated carrots

1/4 cup fresh sliced mushrooms

1 tablespoon vinaigrette dressing (Recipe at the end of this day's plan)

Half cup cooked corn

Half cup canned pears

Recipe of Vegetarian Spaghetti Sauce

2 tablespoon olive oil

2 medium sized tomatoes, chopped

2 small onions, chopped

1 cups sliced zucchini

3 cloves garlic, chopped

1 tablespoon dried oregano

1 tablespoon dried basil

8 oz tomato sauce

6 oz low sodium tomato paste

1 cup water

1. Heat Olive oil in a pan over medium heat. Stir fry onions, garlic and zucchini for five minutes.

2. Add the remaining ingredients.

3. Cover the pan and let it simmer for 45 minutes.

Recipe of the Vinaigrette Dressing

1 full bulb of garlic, peeled and separated

1 tablespoon red wine vinegar

1/4 teaspoon honey

1 tablespoon virgin olive oil

1/4 tsp black pepper

Half cup water

1. Boil garlic cloves in a saucepan.

2. Bring the water to boil and then let it simmer for 15 -20 minutes (until the half cup water is reduced to 2 tablespoon)

3. Turn off the heat, mash the garlic with a spoon and add the remaining ingredients.

Final Words

If you are still not convinced about the effectiveness and benefits of DASH diet, then try it out yourself and be your own judge. 7 days is not a longer time, especially when it comes to your health. Try the 7 day DASH diet plan and feel the difference.

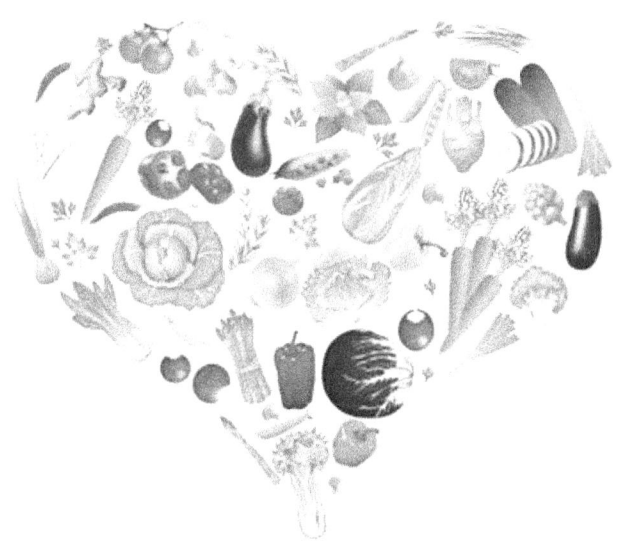

DASH diet has received innumerable praises by the medical experts. It is the best form diet especially for people having hypertension. The little efforts required in getting used to the new eating habits are worth your health and of your loved ones.

DASH Lifestyle! Healthy Lifestyle!

www.ingramcontent.com/pod-product-compliance
Lightning Source LLC
Chambersburg PA
CBHW080341290526
45791CB00009BA/2682